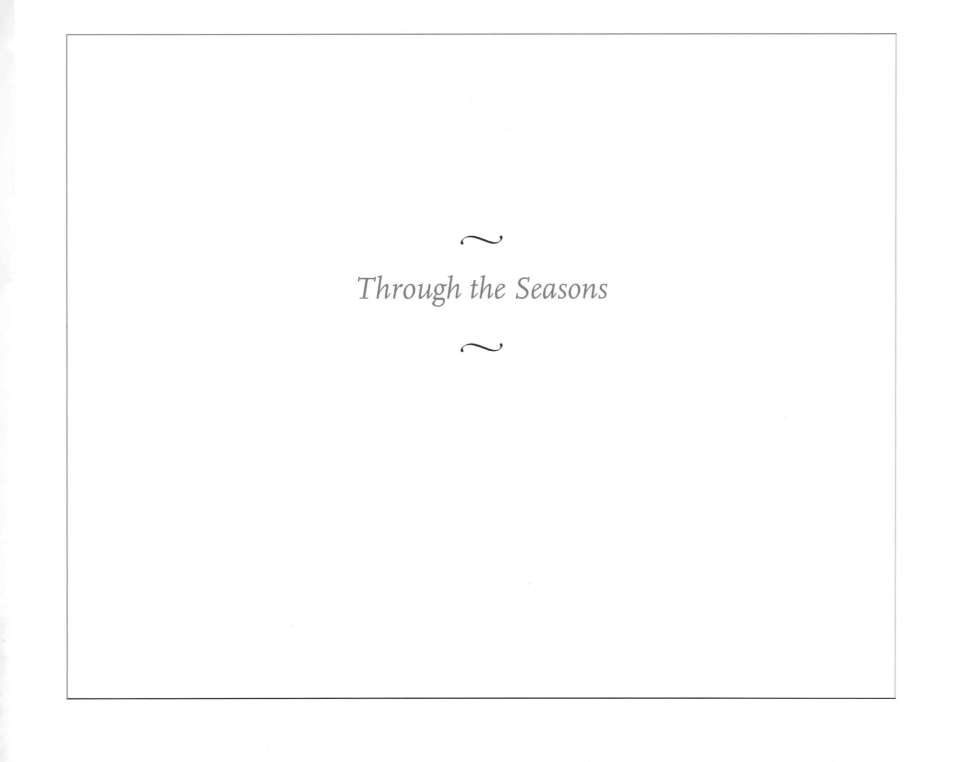

~

Through the Seasons

~

AN ACTIVITY BOOK FOR MEMORY-CHALLENGED ADULTS AND CAREGIVERS

THROUGH
the
SEASONS

CYNTHIA R. GREEN, PH.D. AND JOAN BELOFF, ACC, ALA

The Johns Hopkins University Press
2715 North Charles Street
Baltimore, Maryland 21218-4363
www.press.jhu.edu

PICTURE CREDITS: The photograph on p. 15 is by Zachary Jablons and is used by permission of the photographer. The photographs on pp. 3, 9, 19, 27 are used by permission of Can Stock Photo, Inc. The remaining photographs are used by permission of iStockphoto and are copyrighted by iStockphoto.com and the respective photographer: p. 5, Hedda Gjerpen; p. 7, Nancy Catherine Walker; p. 13, Jalo Porkkala; p. 17, Brian McEntire; p. 23, Kriss Russell; p. 25, Viktor Kitaykin; p. 29, Doug Webb; p. 33, Daniela Andreea Spyropoulos; p. 35, Christine Balderas; p. 37, Jim DeLillo; p. 39, S. Greg Panosian.

Special discounts are available for bulk purchases of this book. For more information, please contact Special Sales at 410-516-6936 or specialsales@press.jhu.edu.

The Johns Hopkins University Press uses environmentally friendly book materials, including recycled text paper that is composed of at least 30 percent post-consumer waste, whenever possible. All of our book papers are acid-free, and our jackets and covers are printed on paper with recycled content.

LIBRARY OF CONGRESS CATALOGING-IN-PUBLICATION DATA

Green, Cynthia R.
    Through the seasons : an activity book for memory-challenged adults and caregivers / Cynthia R. Green, Joan Beloff.
        p.   cm.
    ISBN-13: 978-0-8018-8844-1 (hardcover : alk. paper)
    ISBN-10: 0-8018-8844-1 (hardcover : alk. paper)
        1. Memory disorders—Patients—Rehabilitation. 2. Dementia—Patients—Rehabilitation. 3. Memory disorders in old age—Patients—Rehabilitation. 4. Caregivers. I. Beloff, Joan, 1953– II. Title.
    RC394.M46G74 2008
    362.196'83—dc22   2007039624

A catalog record for this book is available from the British Library.

This book is dedicated to all caregivers who have struggled

to find ways to engage a memory-challenged loved one in meaningful activities.

We hope that it will provide you with the resources to share fond memories

and create new ways to spend quality time together.

~

We thank our families for their love and

for being our constant cheerleaders in this endeavor.

~ CONTENTS ~

INTRODUCTION

Caring for someone with a memory disorder can be an overwhelmingly hard job. As professionals who work with memory-challenged adults and their caregivers, we have witnessed the seemingly unending struggle of our patients and their families to stay connected, engaged, and active in the face of the changes that result from memory-damaging conditions and their progression. This task is often quite daunting.

Memory disorders take a toll on how well affected persons can communicate their thoughts and feelings. The memory-challenged individual may become increasingly unable to share in conversation around the dinner table, at family events, or at social happenings. These communication challenges can lead to isolation from family and friends, social withdrawal, and frustration. In turn, these difficulties can diminish the individual's sense of his or her own value and worth. Activities that the person previously enjoyed can become too difficult for them to pursue independently. Families often share that it is hard to find activities that keep their loved one busy and occupied in a way that feels meaningful. Someone who loved to cook, for example,

may no longer be able to follow the steps of a recipe, or there may be concern about their safety when cooking on their own.

Current research shows that memory-challenged individuals can benefit from continued mental stimulation, even in the face of disease progression. As a result, more and more caregivers, both family members and professionals, have asked: What kind of things can we do to keep our loved one or our clients mentally active and engaged?

Through the Seasons: An Activity Book for Memory-Challenged Adults and Their Caregivers offers a program that takes on these issues. Based on both our own experiences and what we have learned over the years from our clients and their families, we have developed an approach specifically for those affected by memory loss and their families.

- *Through the Seasons* helps maintain communication by increasing opportunities for conversation and dialogue between affected individuals and their caregivers. The book is intended to help family members spend some quality time together, talk about past experiences, and share stories from the past that can become treasured family memories. We have designed it so that even a school-aged child can pore over it with an affected grandparent, sharing an intimacy that is often disrupted by memory loss.

• The program encourages interaction and engagement by providing a variety of meaningful activities that can be shared by memory-challenged persons and their caregivers, whether family members or professionals. The suggested activities are varied and include art, cooking, singing, and scrapbooking. Physical activities are an important aspect of the program, and we encourage their inclusion as much as possible when exploring the experiences. Physical activity helps the individual maintain range of motion, mobility, and circulation. Staying physically active can improve sleep, reduce tension and may decrease wandering. Walking with someone is a good way to promote physical exercise. Of course, you should always check with your and the affected person's physician before participating in a physical activity. Many individuals have past interests, like craft work or performing in singing groups or plays, that can be rekindled.

• This book and its activities are accessible to nonprofessionals and adaptable for use by the senior care professional, either one-to-one or with a larger group. We have included activities that will also boost the affected individual's self-esteem, give a feeling of independence and a sense of success in accomplishing a task.

• *Through the Seasons* provides a source of intellectual stimulation and mental activity, an increasingly important aspect of caring for the memory-challenged individual, whether at home or in a professional setting. It encourages participation in activities that are mentally engaging and intellectually stimulat-

ing for the memory-challenged individual across various degrees of impairment. The conversation prompts and suggested activities purposely range widely, so that individuals and their families can use the program from the early-late to moderate-late stages of disease.

In *Through the Seasons*, you will find a series of simple, common experiences to explore together. These experiences are grouped into four themes, each focusing on a season of the year (fall, winter, spring, summer). The book uses an enriched, multisensory approach, so that the experiences are explored using all five senses (touch, smell, taste, hearing, and vision). Often a nonverbal approach, such as listening or singing familiar songs or smelling familiar foods or spices, can help draw out long-term memories that may otherwise be difficult to share. We have chosen a variety of multisensory activities that work well with the memory-challenged person.

Each experience in *Through the Seasons* offers:

• a beautiful photograph that illustrates the experience and stimulates thoughts, feelings, and memories about it. For example, in the "Summer" section, you will find the experience of eating ice cream, a common and popular summer activity.

• some simple text to begin conversation about the experience, such as, "Ice cream tastes good on a summer day."

• a section on the facing page entitled "Let's Talk About . . . ," where you will find a series of questions to foster further discussion and exploration together. For example, as part of the summer experience featuring ice cream, you might talk about favorite ice cream treats from childhood.

- a section entitled "Let's Try . . . ," with suggested activities to enrich the experience and provide further intellectual stimulation. For the ice cream experience, these activities include having an old-fashioned ice cream party with family and friends and taking a trip to a local ice cream store.

We suggest that, in using this book, the caregiver first look through the entire book and get a sense of what it contains. The program herein can be used in many ways, offering tremendous flexibility in what you can do. For example, you may wish to read the whole book, using only the "Let's Talk About . . . " section to foster conversation. Or you may prefer to begin slowly, starting with the experiences that reflect the current season of the year. Alternatively, you can focus on just one experience, delving deeply into it using several of the suggested activities. These decisions will depend on the stamina of your loved one or client, the setting in which you are using the program, and the time you have to devote to the exploration. We hope that you will use the book in all these different ways, adapting it to include any individual needs of the memory-challenged person or additional activity ideas the experiences suggest to you.

Here are some practical tips and strategies for using *Through the Seasons* that we hope will be helpful in making the program successful for you and your loved one or client:

ESTABLISHING THE SETTING

When using this book, minimize the distractions in the surrounding environment. Find a place that is quiet, where you are unlikely to be interrupted. Memory-challenged individuals often have difficulty maintaining focus and concentration. A quiet setting will increase your chances of engaging in meaningful conversation and sharing in a successful experience.

USING THE BOOK'S FORMAT

Through the Seasons is formatted as a large book that two people can look at together. Physical contact and closeness can be reassuring when someone is struggling with memory loss. Try sitting side by side as you look at the book together. Make frequent eye contact with the memory-challenged person to help him or her stay focused on the task. You can also use nonverbal cues, such as a gentle touch or pointing to details in the photographs to help guide discussion and give direction. Sometimes holding hands, hugging, and other nonverbal interactions will get the person to respond when nothing else seems to be working.

TIPS FOR SUCCESSFUL COMMUNICATION

When a person has difficulty with communication, he or she can become frustrated, angry, depressed, and defensive. Sometimes it appears that the individual is uncooperative, when really he or she cannot understand what you are trying to say. As a guide for enhancing your communications with the affected individual, keep in mind the "three Cs." First, stay *calm* in your actions. In using a steady, reassuring voice, you will set a welcoming and reassuring tone for the interaction. Keep in mind always that the feelings expressed in your voice are as important as the words you say, so try to maintain this sense of calm even when things may not be going exactly as you would like. Next, be *concise* as you speak, using simple words that are concrete and easy to understand. Keep your sentences short and direct, so that they will be easily grasped and followed. Finally, be *consistent* in your choice of words and directions. Using the same phrasing throughout your communications can make it easier for the memory-challenged individual to understand your intent and engage in the conversation. For example, when using the "Let's Talk More About . . . " questions, speak clearly and distinctly in a level and composed manner and keep your wording straightforward. Try to avoid pronouns: instead of saying, "Here it is," point and say, "Here is the turkey in the picture." Ask only one question at a time, making sure to give the person plenty of time to respond. Do not rush the person, as doing so will only add to the confusion and lead to frustration for everyone. If he or she does not seem to understand, repeat the question using the same wording. If after a few minutes this still does not work, try to re-phrase the question slightly. Above all, remember it is important that you be attentive and a good listener. Try not to interrupt the person's thought process, unless it is just to comment on the topic.

Over time, you may find that there will be changes in the way your loved one or client expresses him- or herself and how well the person is able to understand language. It is not uncommon for someone to use familiar words over and over again, to invent new words to describe common objects, or to have difficulty putting words in the correct sequence. The person might revert to his or her native language or at times seem to be speaking nonsense. Again, if you remain calm, concise and consistent in your approach and conversation, it will give both of you a better chance to engage in and benefit from the program.

If you pose a question and you do not understand the response, try to see the meaning or the emotion behind what is being said. Repeating what was said can often lead to clarification. After repeating, you might want to ask some questions to help your loved one or client express what he or she is feeling. The individual's tone of voice or other actions might help you understand what he or she is saying. Try using questions that begin with the words "who," "what," "when," "where," and "how."

USING THE ACTIVITIES

The creative activities that are suggested in this book provide an opportunity for self-expression and increased sense of self-worth. However, people who have memory loss will vary in their ability to participate in activities. In addition, the kinds of activity they can stay engaged with will change as the condition progresses. At later stages, even simple activities that were easily accomplished at a previous time can be a challenge to complete. For that reason, we have provided a wide variety of activities that range in approach and difficulty. Choose what seems to fit the person's current abilities.

How can you successfully use these activities across the different stages of memory loss? First, remember to allow your loved one to be as independent as possible during the activity. Do not be concerned with the outcome of the exercise. For example, if you are making a crafts project, do not worry if the pieces are not put together properly or the item is not painted correctly. It is more important to spend quality time together than to have a perfectly finished product. Interrupting the process to straighten up a photograph or correcting minor lyrics of a song may diminish the memory-challenged person's sense of accomplishment or self-worth.

Second, adapt the activities as necessary. Sometimes you might need to break down the steps of the activity to make it easier to accomplish. For example, you might need to take several days to do an activity such as scrapbooking, cutting out photographs on one day and gluing them into the book on the next. Or you may need to modify certain aspects of an activity to meet the special needs of your loved one or client. For example, an individual who uses a wheelchair may not be able to take a walk through the grass. However, he or she will be able to feel blades of grass brushed against his or her cheek, or even across his or her feet.

Set appropriate expectations for what you are trying to accomplish. Be realistic about what the memory-challenged individual can accomplish. If you attempt activities that are too difficult, you will both feel frustrated and disappointed. Likewise, activities that are overly simple may feel demeaning and disappointing. Also keep in mind that people with memory loss are still people! Like you, they will have personal preferences about which activities they like and dislike. Try to select activities that you know they might have enjoyed previously. While you might encourage your loved one or client to try something new, do not force the participation. Everyone will benefit most fully from this program if the memory-challenged individual is met at his or her level of ability and interest.

ENCOURAGING REMINISCENCE

Many of the activities included in *Through the Seasons* can help the individual tap into memories that are still alive to him or her.

In most memory disorders, long-term memories such as those about childhood or early adulthood remain accessible and well preserved into even some of the later stages of illness. Reminiscing allows the individual an opportunity to reflect on and feel good about the contributions that he or she made during his or her lifetime. It also is a wonderful opportunity for younger family members or newly acquainted caregivers to learn more about the caregiver's past history, traditions, and accomplishments. The experiences and activities included here are designed to encourage reminiscing, and we suggest that you look for opportunities to take advantage of this whenever possible. For example, when making memory boxes or scrapbooks try to use personal articles that hold sentimental value. This will help stimulate the conversation and prompt the individual to talk about stories and special memories from the past. Try to keep a diary of the stories and memories that are shared. As memory declines further, it will become increasingly difficult for your loved one or client to connect with those memories; you can use the diary to explore and share those stories again, which may be comforting and encourage conversation. You can look back on those stories and share them again with your loved one or client, continuing in that way to explore with the person even as the disease progresses. The diary can also serve as a wonderful way to preserve the affected individual's stories and memories for the future.

KEEPING IT SAFE

Whenever you engage a memory-challenged adult in an activity, you must include an assessment of any safety issues that such participation may raise. Memory disorders often can affect an individual's judgment about his or her own safety and ability. Therefore, you must take responsibility for making sound decisions and taking precautions to ensure that the person can safely participate in any planned activity. Before introducing an activity, take a good look at any safety challenges it may raise. For example, can the person safely perform the physical activity that is required, such as walking across a lawn or cutting up apples? What steps will you need to take to ensure that the person is protected from accidents while cooking or using scissors? If you are preparing for a gathering of several persons, such as an ice cream social, are there dietary restrictions to consider? Once you have reviewed all the possible safety issues associated with an activity, think through how you can modify or adjust the activity to make it safe. For example, you may need to preslice apples for an applesauce-making activity or provide sugar-free ice cream and toppings if many of the persons attending your ice cream social follow a sugar-free diet.

DEALING WITH FRUSTRATION

There may be times in using *Through the Seasons* when the memory-challenged individual becomes frustrated, withdrawn, or even agitated. If you see the person growing irritated, try to understand what is causing the individual to become angry or upset. Think about what happened before the person became upset and try to identify what might have triggered the reaction. Sometimes he or she might not feel like doing something, just as you yourself might feel on certain days. Other times it might be that he or she is unable to express another need, such as having to go to the bathroom or wanting something to drink. Try to address the problem then and see if you can go on with the discussion or activity. If the person continues to be upset or becomes uncooperative, stop the project and try again later. Always be positive and reassuring and speak in a soft, slow tone. If needed, use music or touch to help calm the individual before you move away to something else. Keeping the interactions positive and enjoyable will benefit everyone.

WE HOPE THAT *Through the Seasons* will bring many wonderful shared experiences to the lives of memory-challenged individuals and those who care for them. It is our sincerest wish that this book will make a difference, not only in stimulating old memories but also in creating new ones. We look forward to hearing the many ways in which you use this book and make the experiences and activities your own. Thank you for letting us be part of your caring process.

Through the Seasons

FALL

LET'S TALK ABOUT . . .

- What is your favorite food to eat on Thanksgiving Day? Are there special foods your family eats on Thanksgiving?

- What kind of pie do you like to eat on Thanksgiving?

- Do you have a special recipe for stuffing?

- Who would come to your home for Thanksgiving dinner?

- Do you have special family traditions for Thanksgiving, such as a special song or prayer?

- What are you thankful for?

LET'S TRY . . .

- Cooking some Thanksgiving foods, such as a turkey, stuffing, or roasted chestnuts.

- Making cranberry sauce.

- Creating a Thanksgiving scrapbook using photographs or images from magazines or old cookbooks.

- Decorating an orange with cloves, then putting it on a string and hanging it up in the room.

- Singing Thanksgiving songs, such as "We Gather Together," "The Turkey Ran Away," etc.

- Creating a Thanksgiving family book, using old family recipes, photographs, and stories from your loved one's past (which may need to be dictated to you). Share the book with other family members.

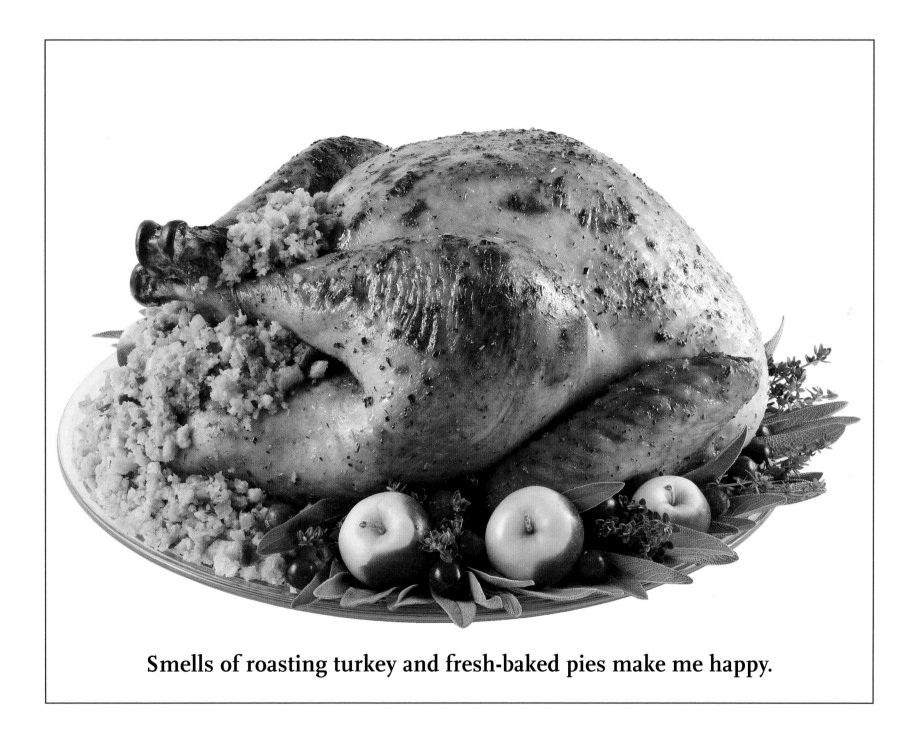

Smells of roasting turkey and fresh-baked pies make me happy.

LET'S TALK ABOUT . . .

- Did you ever go apple picking? Where would you go to pick apples?

- Did you ever smell apples baking or cooking on the stovetop?

- Did you ever make applesauce?

- What do apples make you think about?

- Did you have an apple tree in your yard? in your neighborhood?

- Apples can be sweet or tart, crunchy or soft. What different apple tastes do you like?

- Many traditions have special recipes that use apples. What family recipes do you have that use apples?

LET'S TRY . . .

- Making an apple crisp or an apple pie.

- Making applesauce. You can either make the applesauce from scratch using a recipe from a cookbook or warm ready-made applesauce on the stovetop, adding spices such as cinnamon and clove.

- Visiting a local farm to walk through the orchards and pick apples.

- Going to the grocery store or a farmer's market to look at the different kinds of apples.

- Cutting and eating apples, dipping them in honey or chocolate. Listen to the crunchy sounds as you eat the apples.

- Drinking apple cider. You can make mulled cider by heating the cider with mulling spices (which you can purchase at the grocery store).

- Singing "Don't Sit under the Apple Tree."

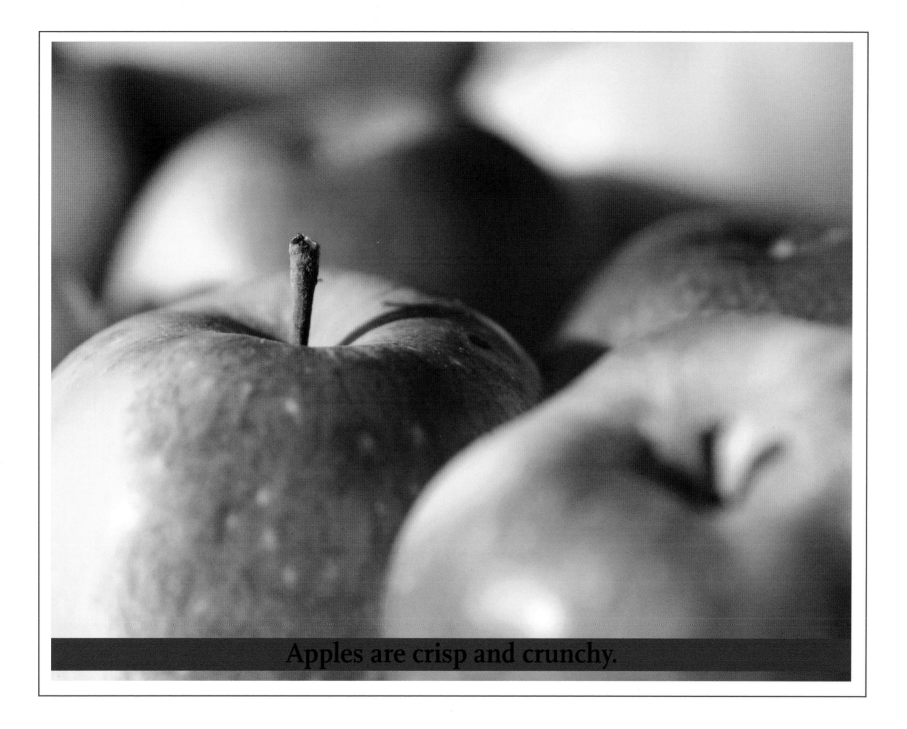

Apples are crisp and crunchy.

LET'S TALK ABOUT . . .

- What was your favorite Halloween costume?

- What is your favorite candy?

- Did you ever carve a pumpkin on Halloween, or make a jack-o'-lantern?

- Did you ever roast pumpkin seeds?

- Did you ever bob for apples?

- What traditions did your family have for Halloween?

- Did you ever dress up in a costume for other holidays or special events?

LET'S TRY . . .

- Carving or painting a pumpkin.

- Making pumpkin treats, such as pumpkin bread or pumpkin muffins. You can make cookies shaped as pumpkins and decorate them as jack-o'-lanterns with orange and black icing.

- Roasting and eating pumpkin seeds.

- Having a Halloween party for family and friends. You can make Halloween hats out of plain party hats decorated with Halloween-themed stickers. Decorate the room with Halloween decorations, and then share different kinds of Halloween candy, mulled cider, and other Halloween treats. (You can find the art supplies at a crafts store.)

- Making a Halloween scrapbook using pictures and illustrations from magazines and catalogues.

- Putting together bags of candy to give to children for Halloween. You can decorate the bags using markers and stickers.

- Listening to Halloween music.

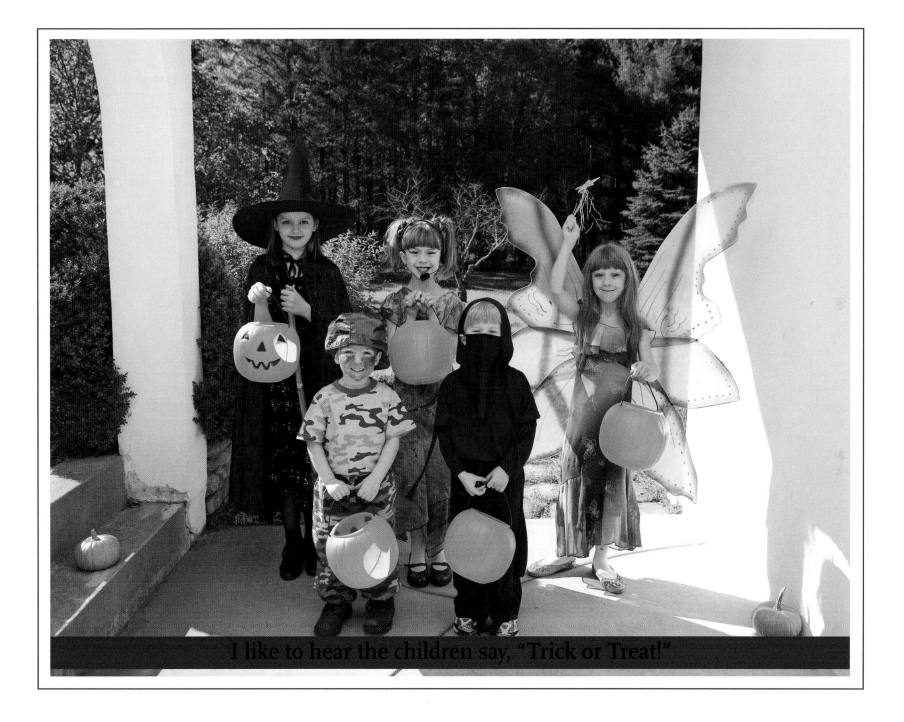

I like to hear the children say, "Trick or Treat!"

LET'S TALK ABOUT . . .

- Do you ever sit and watch the leaves fall from the trees?

- Do you like to rake leaves?

- What kind of games would you play in the fallen leaves?

- What do the smells of fall remind you of?

- Do you remember the smell of leaves burning?

- What are your favorite fall colors?

LET'S TRY . . .

- Taking a drive to see the fall foliage.

- Collecting leaves and making a collage.

- Raking leaves.

- Taking a walk outside to look at the leaves and talk about what season it is, how the leaves look, and how they will change next.

- Walking through leaves, kicking through them, or throwing them up in the air and watching as they fall.

- Making cookies in the shape of leaves, decorating them with icing in fall colors.

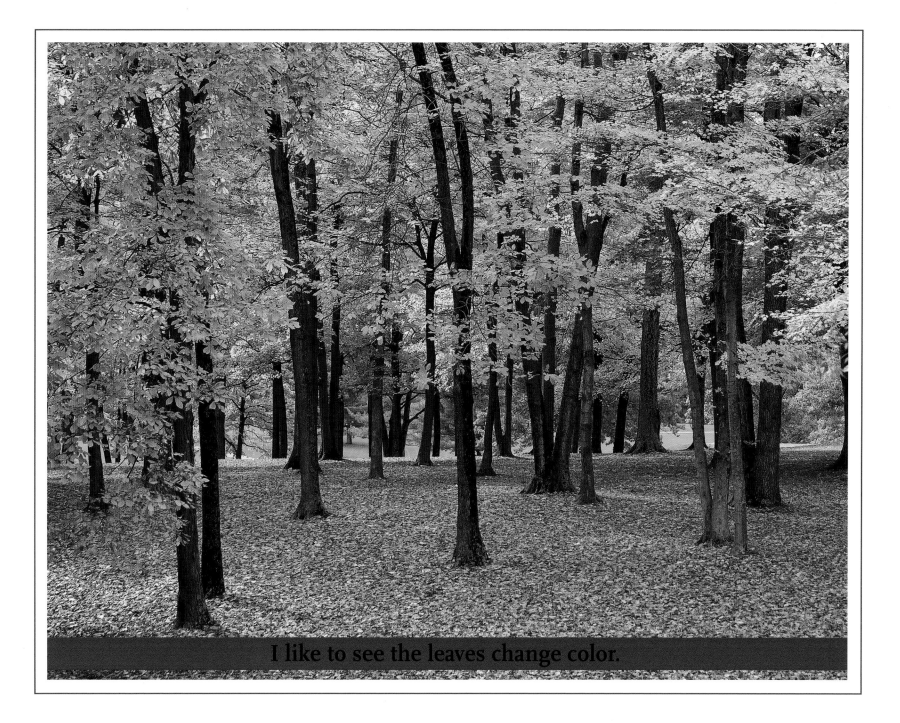

I like to see the leaves change color.

SUMMER

FALL

WINTER

SPRING

SUMMER

FALL

LET'S TALK ABOUT . . .

- Did you ever build a snowman?

- Did you like to go sledding?

- What games did you play in the snow?

- Do you remember a big snowstorm when you were young?

- Did you like sports in the winter, such as skiing or ice skating?

- Do you like to eat hot soup on a snowy day? What is your favorite kind of soup?

LET'S TRY . . .

- Shaking snow globes to watch the snow fall.

- Cutting out paper snowflakes from a doily.

- Making snowmen by gluing together white foam balls and decorating them with stickers and markers. (You can find these supplies at a crafts store.)

- Singing songs about snow, such as "Let it Snow" or "Jingle Bells."

- Making "snow" by scraping ice, then feeling the texture and cold.

- Eating a "snow cone" by making a treat out of crushed ice and fruit juice.

- Taking a walk in the snow.

- Going for a sleigh ride.

- Making a pot of soup and eating together.

- Making a scrapbook using pictures of winter scenes, winter clothing, and other things from wintertime.

- Writing down some favorite wintertime recollections from childhood, such as stories about a favorite sledding hill, family winter activities, family recipes, or special holiday memories. Share these stories with other family members.

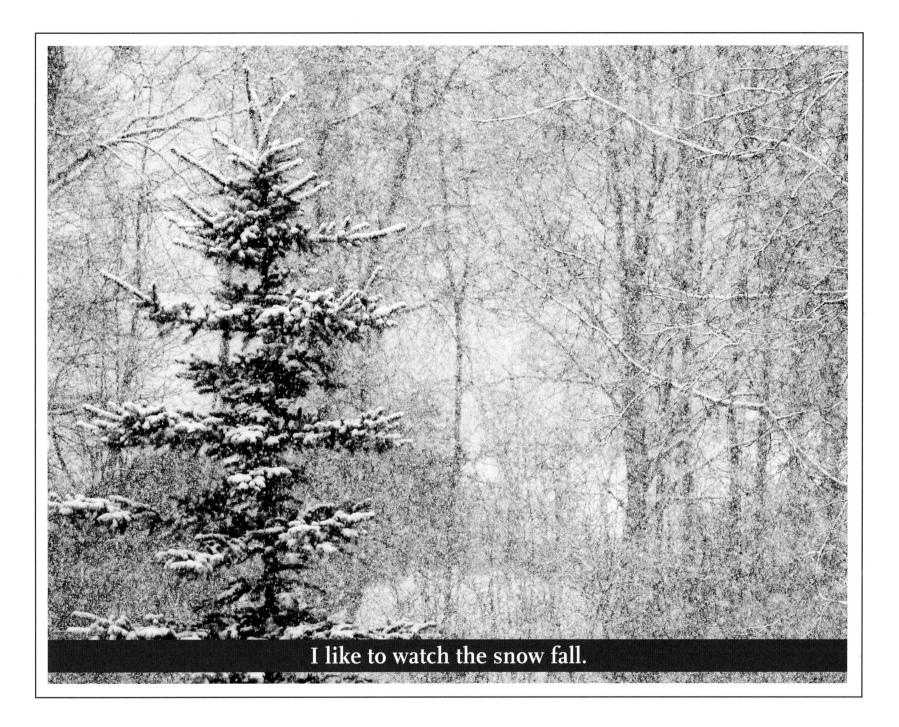

I like to watch the snow fall.

LET'S TALK ABOUT . . .

- Do you have a favorite blanket? What color is it?

- Do you like to sleep in a cold room or a warm room?

- Do you remember your favorite childhood blanket?

- Do you like to be wrapped up in a blanket?

- Did you ever sit under a blanket in front of a roaring fire?

- Did you ever wrap a baby in a blanket?

LET'S TRY . . .

- Touching different kinds of blanket materials, such as wool, cotton, and fleece, and talking about how they feel.

- Snuggling together under a big blanket or quilt.

- Wrapping a baby doll in a blanket.

- Making a blanket by cutting large pieces of flannel or fleece and sewing them together.

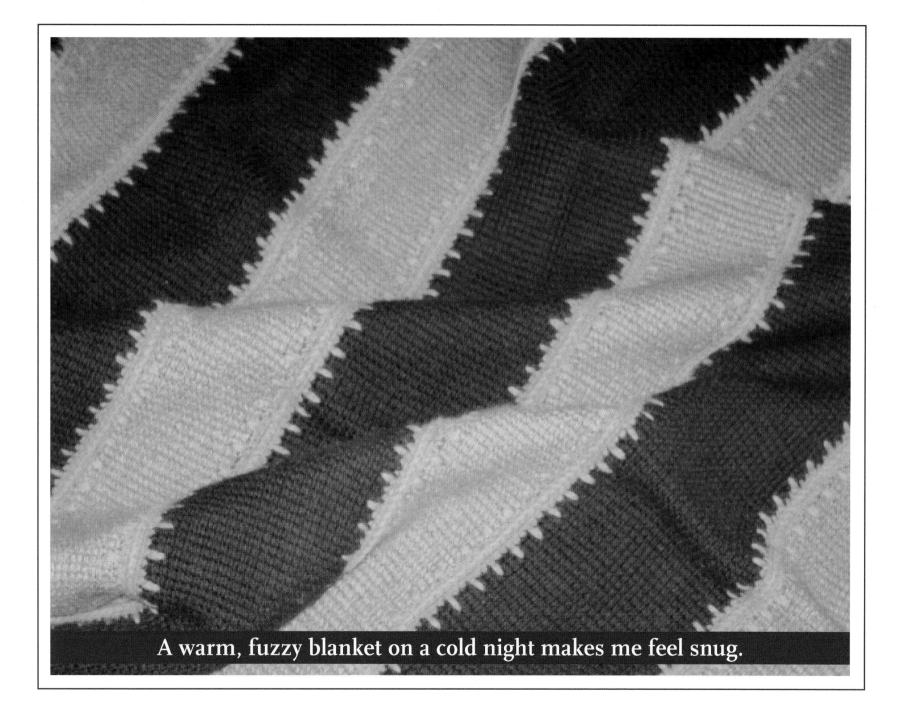

A warm, fuzzy blanket on a cold night makes me feel snug.

LET'S TALK ABOUT . . .

- Do you like to drink hot chocolate when it is cold outside?

- What does hot chocolate remind you of?

- How did you make your hot chocolate? Did you use milk or water? Was it sweet? spicy? Did you put anything on top?

- Does sipping hot chocolate make you feel warm inside?

- Do you like to drink hot chocolate in a mug? in a glass?

- What do you like to eat with your hot chocolate?

LET'S TRY . . .

- Drinking hot chocolate made from a mix.

- Making hot chocolate from scratch, by melting chocolate and mixing with milk. Add marshmallows or whipped cream if you like.

- Making hot chocolate using recipes from different countries, such as Mexico, France, or Holland.

- Baking cookies to eat with your hot chocolate.

- Decorating mugs to use for hot chocolate. (Mug-making kits are available at most craft stores.)

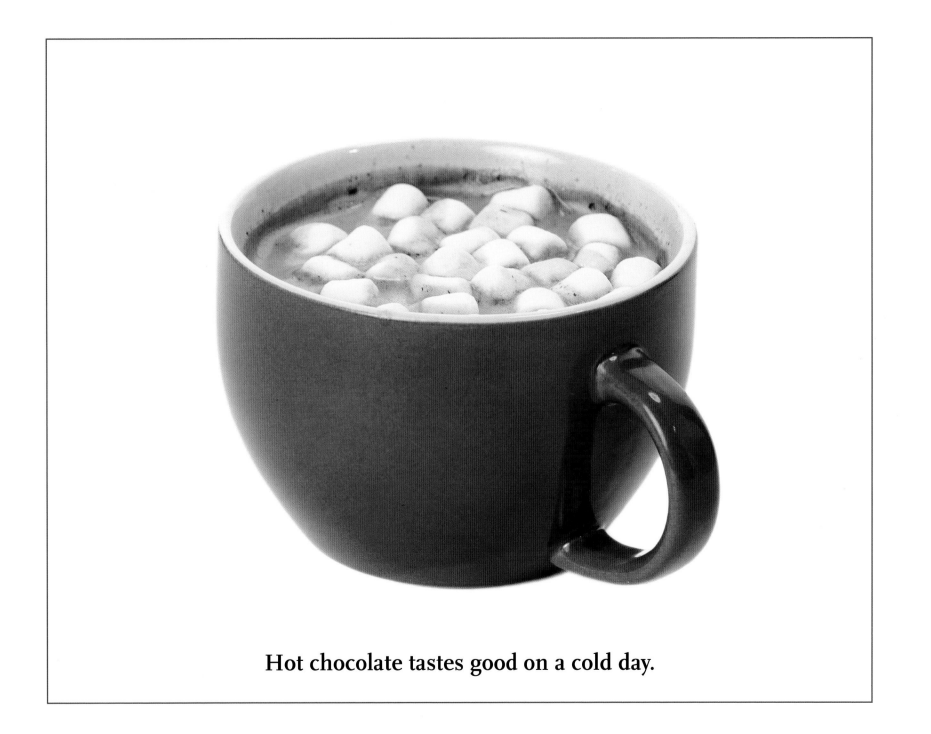

Hot chocolate tastes good on a cold day.

LET'S TALK ABOUT . . .

- What is your favorite kind of cookie?

- Did you ever bake cookies with your mother or grandmother?

- Did you ever bake cookies with children?

- Do you have favorite cookies for Christmas, Hannukah, or Kwanza?

- Did you keep your cookies in a cookie jar?

LET'S TRY . . .

- Baking cookies from premade dough or from scratch.

- Using cookie cutters of different winter theme shapes to make cookies. Decorate them with white frosting and sugar sprinkles.

- Visiting a local bakery together.

- Wrapping cookies to give as gifts.

- Eating your fresh-baked cookies with a favorite drink.

- Making a cookie collage using pictures of cookies from magazines.

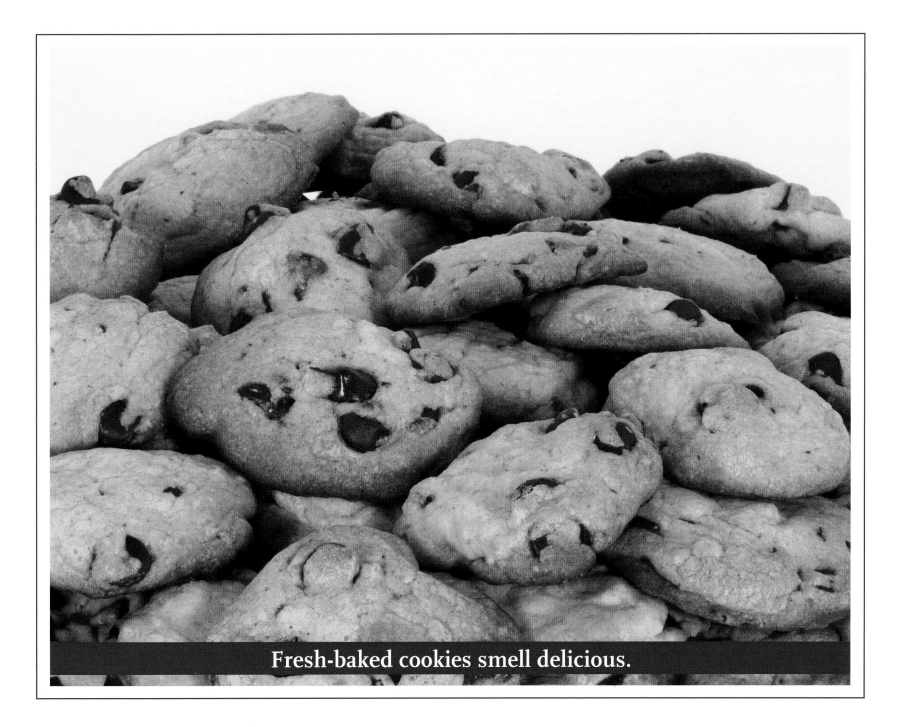

Fresh-baked cookies smell delicious.

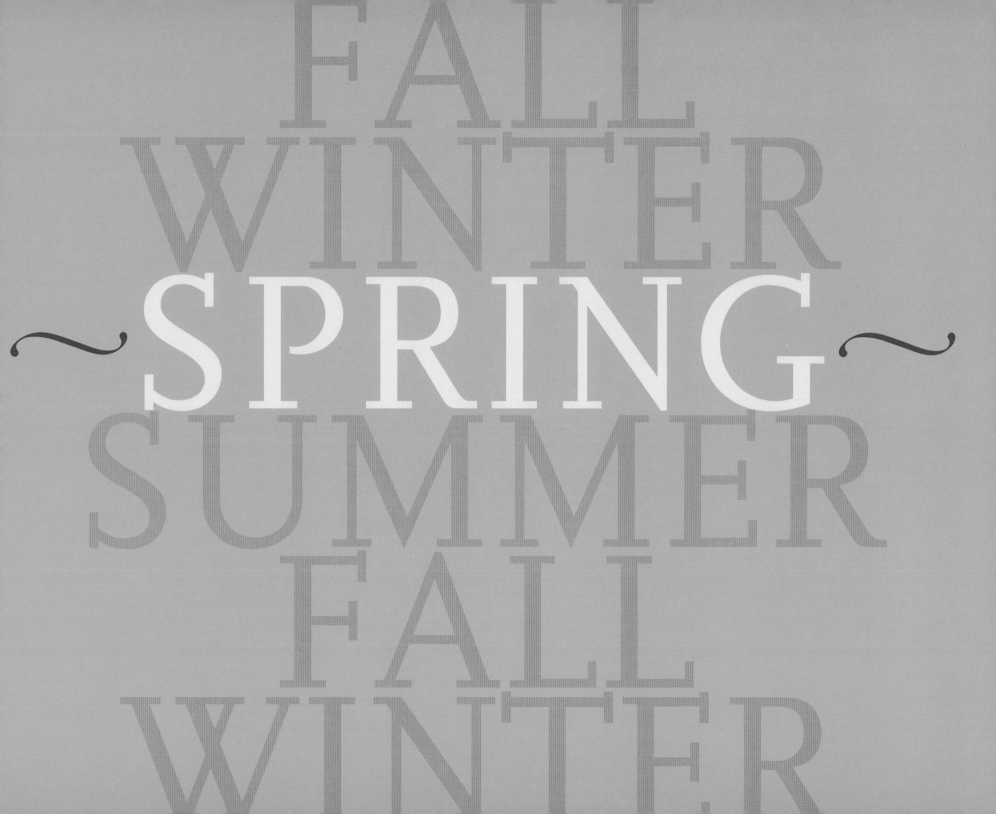

LET'S TALK ABOUT . . .

- Do you remember a very windy day in spring?

- Did you hang your laundry out to dry on windy days?

- Do you like to listen to the sound of wind chimes?

- Do you like to fly a kite on a windy day?

- Did you ever see a wind storm, like a twister or hurricane or sandstorm?

LET'S TRY . . .

- Making a simple kite out of brown paper, craft sticks, fabric strips, and string. You can decorate the kite with stickers and markers. (You can find these supplies at a crafts store.)

- Making a wind indicator out of some long fabric strips and a stick. You can then mount the wind indicator outside a window, using it to see when the wind is blowing.

- Listening to wind chimes. Try wind chimes of different sizes, shapes, and materials, and talk about the difference in their sounds.

- Making wind chimes by tying shells onto a wire loop. (You can find these supplies at a crafts store.)

- Blowing across the top of an open bottle and listening to the sound. You can fill bottles with different amounts of water and try "playing" simple songs, such as "Jack and Jill" and "Row, Row, Row Your Boat," by blowing on the bottles.

- Taking a walk on a windy spring day.

- Playing a parachute game: Take a sheet, grab the sides, and move it up and down to create wind.

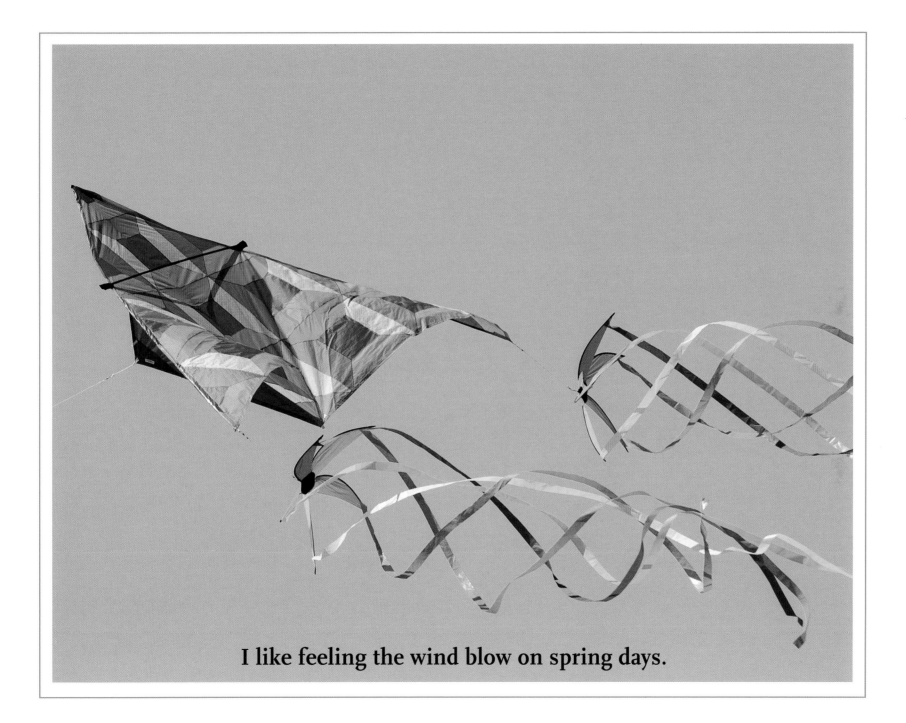

I like feeling the wind blow on spring days.

- What does freshly cut grass smell like to you?

- What does fresh cut grass remind you of?

- Did you ever cut grass when you were younger?

- How does the grass feel when you walk on it barefoot?

- What games would you play in the yard or in the park when you were young?

- Planting grass seeds in a container and growing the grass. You can talk each day about how the grass is growing and about caring for the growing grass.

- Walking across a freshly mowed lawn, if possible with bare feet.

- Playing a game of horseshoes in the grass.

- Having a picnic outside on a grassy lawn.

- Touching the grass and talking about how it feels and smells.

- Going to an outdoor concert and sitting on the grass.

- Making a terrarium using a round fish bowl. Use a variety of colorful plants, which you can find at your local garden center.

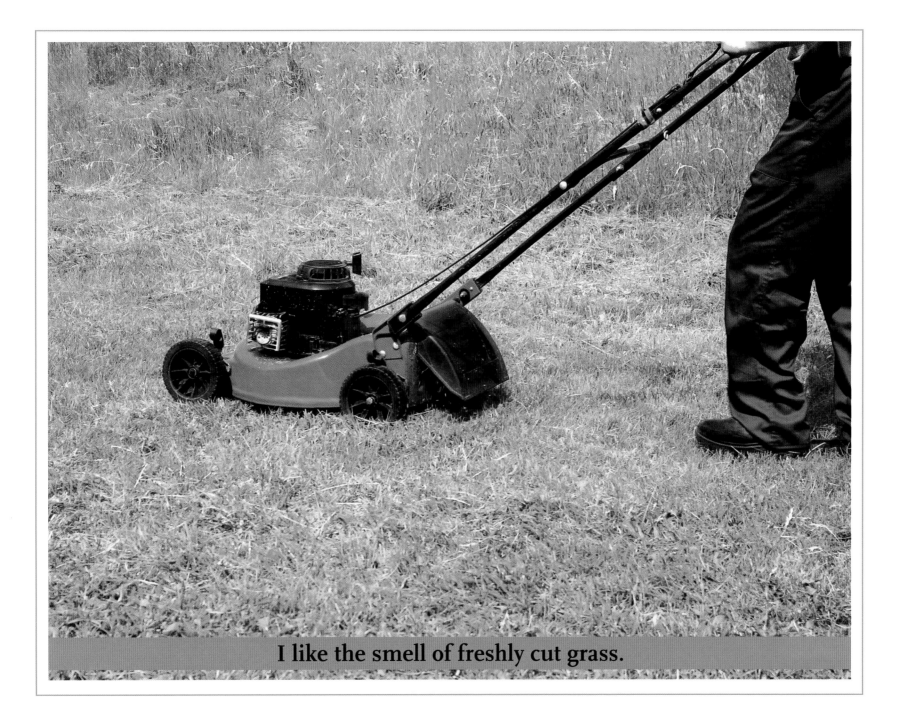

I like the smell of freshly cut grass.

- What are some of your favorite spring flowers? Why do you like them?

- Did you ever plant spring flowers?

- What do flowers in springtime remind you of?

- What color flowers do you like best?

- What flowers have the best smell?

- Where have you seen flower gardens?

- Do you like watching the butterflies fly in springtime?

- Planting spring flower bulbs in a pot or in the garden.

- Smelling different kinds of spring flowers.

- Taking a walk in a spring garden.

- Weeding a flower bed.

- Making a potpourri out of dried flowers. (Mix dried flowers from the craft store, broken into small pieces, in a bowl. Add a few drops of scented oil. Then put the potpourri in sachet bags, small decorative paper boxes, or in a glass bowl for display.)

- Decorating a small cardboard storage box with pictures of spring flowers. You can also use this box for keeping the potpourri.

- Looking at books with photographs of spring flowers.

- Singing songs with names of flowers in them, such as "Daisy, Daisy" and "Tip Toe through the Tulips."

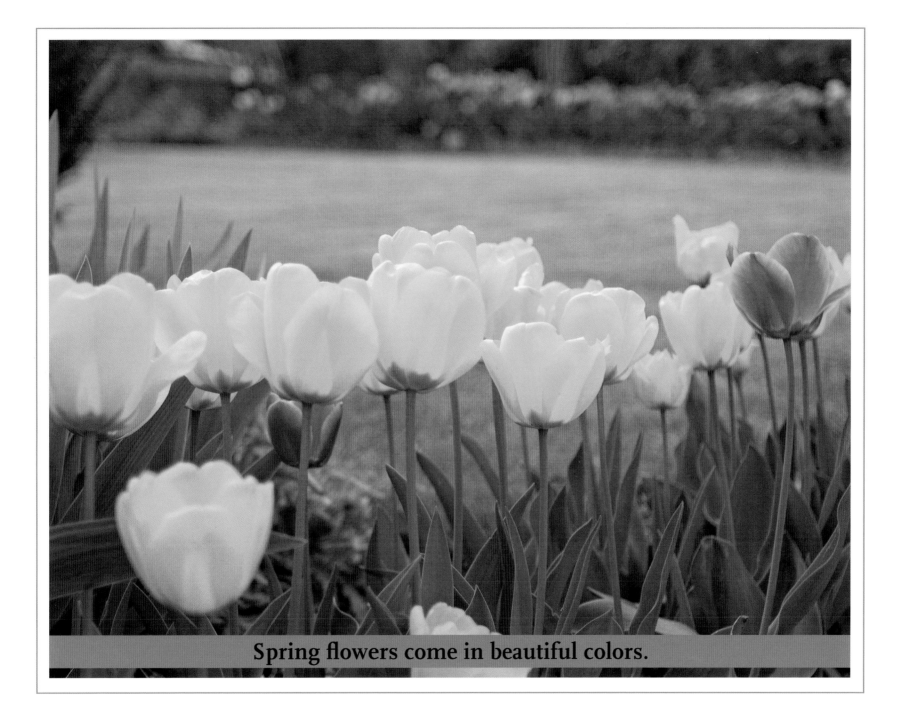

Spring flowers come in beautiful colors.

- What are the different sounds that birds make?

- Can you name some types of birds?

- What is your favorite kind of bird?

- Did you ever have a pet bird? What kind?
  What was its name?

- What does the sound of birds singing in the spring
  make you think of?

- Did you ever see a bird's nest? Could you see the eggs or
  chicks inside?

- Making a bird feeder and hanging it outside the window.
  (You can get bird feeder kits at a crafts store.)

- Stringing pretzels or cereal, such as Cheerios, and
  hanging it outside the window for the birds to eat.

- Putting a large bowl with water outside the window for
  the birds to use as a bird bath.

- Touching feathers and talking about how they feel on
  our hands and face and under our chins.

- Taking a walk in the park or neighborhood looking and
  listening for different types of birds.

- Visiting an aviary.

- Listening to bird calls on a tape.

- Looking at pictures in a bird-watching handbook.

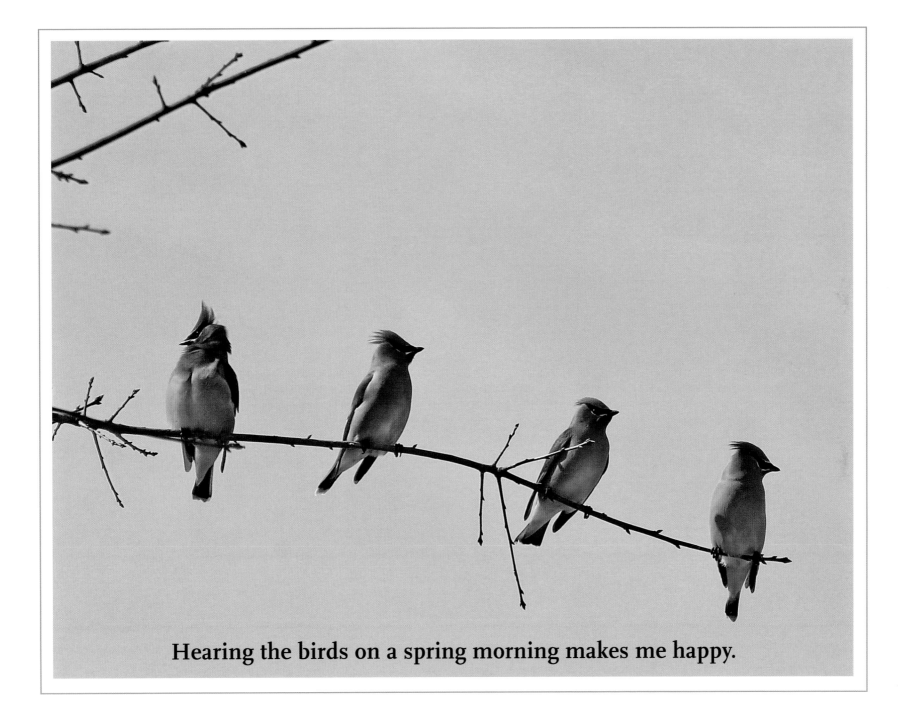

Hearing the birds on a spring morning makes me happy.

SUMMER

LET'S TALK ABOUT . . .

- What did you like to play outside when you were small?

- What sounds do children make when they play?

- How do you feel when you hear children laughing?

- What other sounds do you hear outside in the summer?

LET'S TRY . . .

- Watching children play on a playground.

- Playing some outside games, such as rolling a ball to each other or having a gentle game of catch.

- Having a bean bag toss.

- Watching children play familiar games, such as hopscotch or jacks, and talking about memories of playing them.

- If possible, providing interaction with young children to play some gentle games.

- Swinging gently on an outdoor porch swing.

- If your loved one is still able, encourage him or her to teach a simple game to a grandchild.

- Make a games memory box: Put familiar outdoor game objects, such as balls, jacks, sidewalk chalk, and marbles, in a shoebox. You can use the objects in the box to look at and talk about childhood memories. If you'd like, you can decorate the shoebox using wrapping paper or magazine photos with game playing themes.

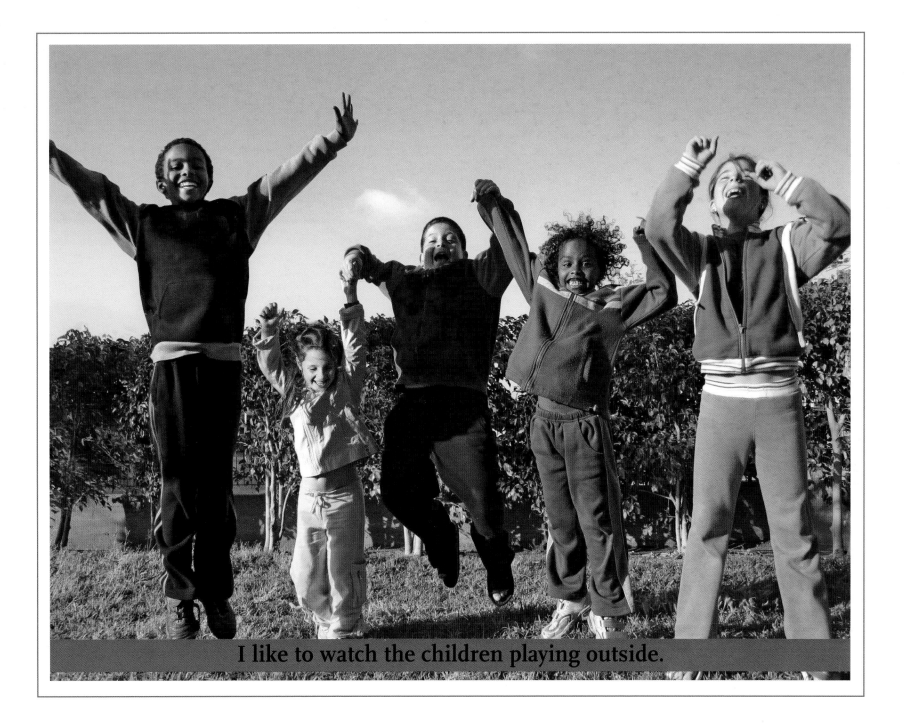

I like to watch the children playing outside.

LET'S TALK ABOUT . . .

- What is your favorite flavor of ice cream?

- Do you like to eat your ice cream from a cone or a cup?

- What are your favorite toppings for ice cream?

- Did you ever make ice cream? How did you do it?

- Where would you eat ice cream in the summer? at the beach? on a porch?

- What are your favorite ice cream treats: ice cream sandwiches, sundaes, banana splits, sodas?

LET'S TRY . . .

- Tasting different flavors of ice cream.

- Making homemade ice cream, an ice cream cake, or freezer popsicles.

- Making homemade whipped cream to eat with your ice cream.

- Making sundaes, banana splits, or ice cream sodas.

- Visiting an ice cream parlor.

- Having an old-fashioned ice cream parlor party with family and friends. (Make old-fashioned ice cream treats, such as malteds, ice cream sodas, and egg creams.)

- Reading some poems about ice cream.

- Singing "Lazy Days of Summer."

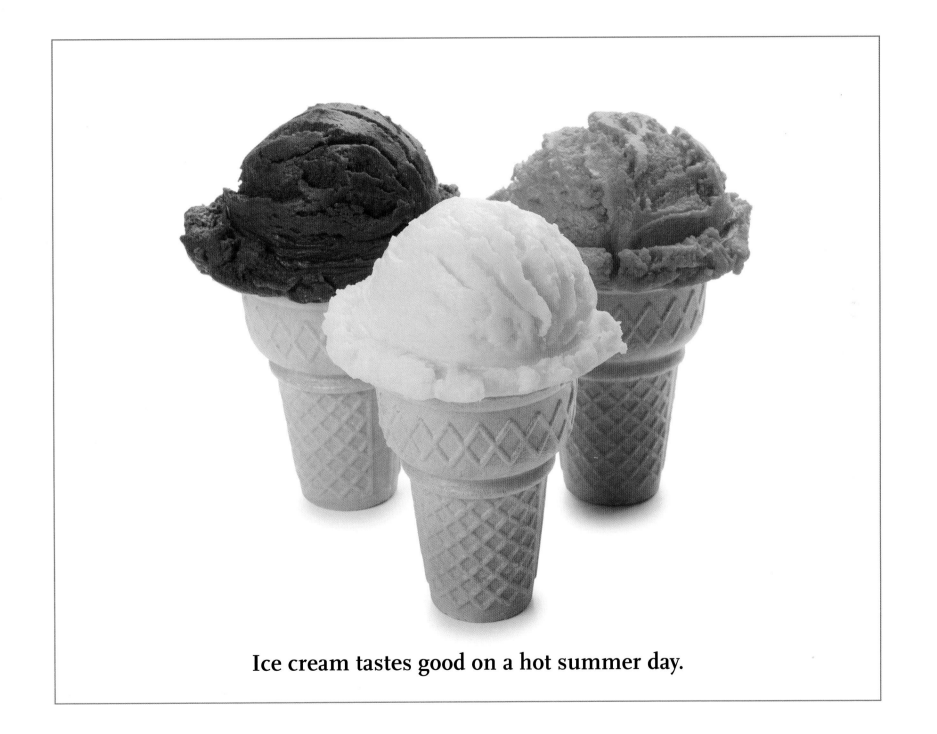

Ice cream tastes good on a hot summer day.

LET'S TALK ABOUT . . .

- What are your favorite foods to barbecue?

- Did your family barbecue in the backyard? at a park? at the beach?

- What other foods do people eat at a barbecue?

- Did you ever have a watermelon seed spitting contest?

- Did you like to roast marshmallows at a barbecue?

LET'S TRY . . .

- Having a barbecue with family and friends.

- Tasting the different condiments used at a barbecue, such as ketchup, mustard, relish, pickles, barbecue sauce.

- Tasting barbecued foods from other cultures, such as Mexico and India.

- Looking at barbecue cookbooks.

- Eating desserts found at barbecues, such as watermelon, fruit salad, and s'mores.

- Making a salad for the barbecue using colorful, seasonal vegetables. Have everything washed and cut up ahead of time, so you can mix the ingredients together.

- Making a potato salad or cole slaw.

- Making a collage using photographs of favorite barbecue foods and backyard scenes.

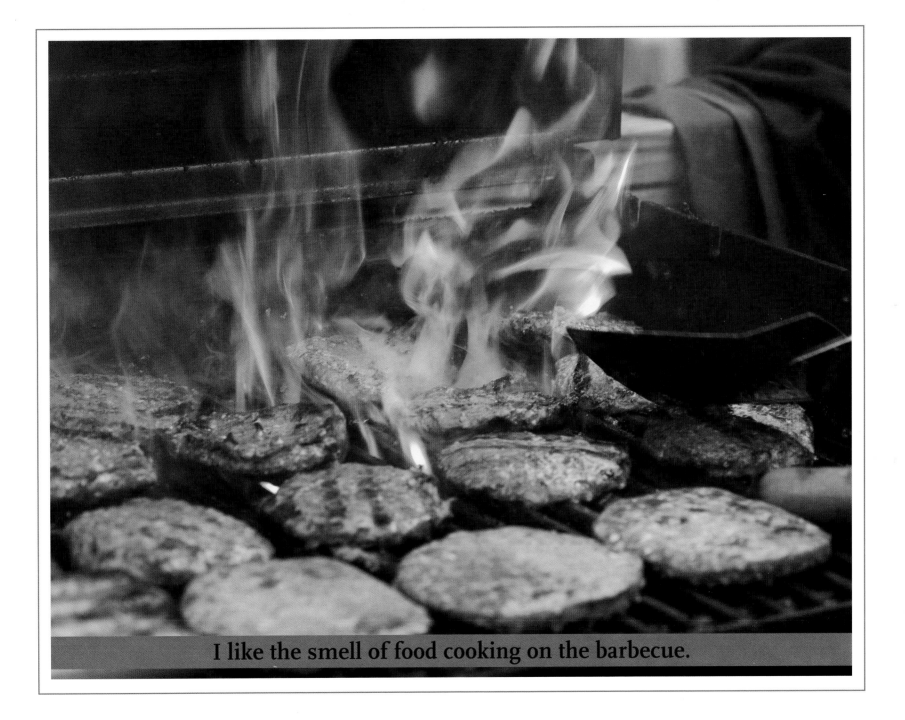

I like the smell of food cooking on the barbecue.

LET'S TALK ABOUT . . .

- Have you visited the beach in summer? Where did you go to the beach?

- What are the sounds we hear at the beach?

- What kinds of things would you find in the sand?

- How does the sand feel on your feet at the beach?

- Do you like to go for walks on the beach?

- Do you like to swim in the ocean?

- What kinds of games would you play at the beach?

- How do the sounds by the ocean make you feel?

LET'S TRY . . .

- Making a sand art project. (You can find sand art project kits at most craft stores.)

- Buying a bag of sand and warming it in the sun. Then try touching the sand, running it through your fingers, putting your bare feet in it. Talk about how it feels.

- Making a keepsake beach box. Use a shoebox or other cardboard box and decorate it with paint, sea shells, or pictures of the seashore cut from magazines. Inside the box, put sand and objects you can find at the beach.

- Listening to a tape or CD of ocean sounds.

- Watching an old movie with a beach theme, such as "Beach Party" or "Beach Blanket Bingo."

- Taking a walk at the beach, either on the sand or on a boardwalk.

- Getting a conch shell and listening to the sounds of the ocean.

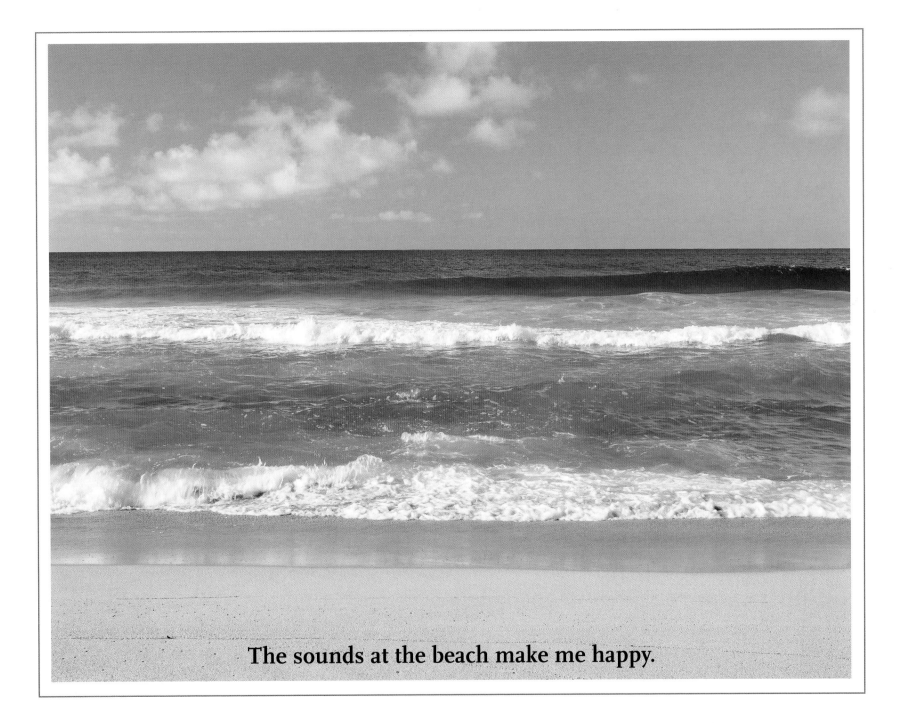

The sounds at the beach make me happy.

RESOURCES FOR CAREGIVERS

ORGANIZATIONS AND ASSOCIATIONS

Numerous organizations and associations offer information for individuals affected by a memory disorder and their families. As a caregiver, you might find it helpful to get information from organizations about caring for someone with a memory disorder, as well as caring for yourself. In addition to information about Alzheimer disease and related memory disorders, several organizations provide supportive services and local resources for individuals who have a memory disorder and for their caregivers. Listed below are several groups through which you can learn more about support groups, services, research, and additional publications.

Alzheimer's Disease Education and Referral (ADEAR) Center

P.O. Box 8250
Silver Spring, MD 20907-8250
800-438-4380
301-495-3334 (fax)
www.alzheimers.nia.nih.gov

Part of the National Institute on Aging, the Alzheimer's Disease Education and Referral (ADEAR) Center is funded by the federal government. It offers information and publications on diagnosis, treatment, patient care, caregiver needs, long-term care, education and training, and research related to Alzheimer disease. The staff respond to telephone and written requests and can make referrals to local and national resources. Publications and videos can be ordered through the ADEAR Center or via their web site.

Alzheimer's Association

225 North Michigan Avenue, Suite 1700
Chicago, IL 60601-7633
800-272-3900
www.alz.org

The Alzheimer's Association is the largest U.S. nonprofit association supporting people with Alzheimer disease and related memory disorders, their families, and caregivers. With almost 300 chapters nationwide, the Alzheimer's Association provides referrals to local resources and services and sponsors support groups and educational programs for memory-challenged individuals and their families. Online and print versions of publications are available at their web site.

The National Institute on Aging Information Center
P.O. Box 8057
Gaithersburg, MD 20898-8057
800-222-2225
800-222-4225 (TTY)
www.nia.nih.gov

The National Institute on Aging Information Center issues a number of publications on healthy aging that are appropriate for both memory-challenged individuals and their caregivers. These include the "Age Page" series and the "NIA Exercise Kit," which offers both an exercise guide and a closed-captioned video. NIA publications can be viewed and ordered via their website at www.nia.nih.gov/HealthInformation/Publications.

National Institute on Aging
Senior Health Website
www.nih.seniorhealth.gov

This senior-friendly website is co-sponsored by the National Institute on Aging and the National Library of Medicine. It offers information on health topics of common concern to older adults.

Administration on Aging
Alzheimer's Resource Room
www.aoa.gov/alzheimers

The Administration on Aging's Alzheimer's Resource Room is an excellent website service for individuals affected by memory disorders and for their families. News regarding the disease, research updates, information about supportive services, and more is available. The website also provides information and links for professionals working with memory-challenged individuals.

Children of Aging Parents
P.O. Box 167
Richboro, PA 18954
800-227-7294
www.caps4caregivers.org

This nonprofit group provides information and materials for adult children caring for their parents. Although the information they provide is not only for caregivers of people with a memory disorder, it can be useful.

Family Caregiver Alliance
180 Montgomery Street, Suite 1100
San Francisco, CA 94104
800-445-8106
www.caregiver.org

The Family Caregiver Alliance is a community-based nonprofit organization offering support services for those caring for adults with Alzheimer disease, stroke, traumatic brain injury, or another cognitive disorder. Programs and services include their Information Clearinghouse for FCA's publications.

Well Spouse Association
63 West Main Street, Suite H
Freehold, NJ 07728
800-838-0879
www.wellspouse.org

Well Spouse is a nonprofit association offering support and information to spouses and partners of chronically ill and/or disabled persons. "Mainstay," the newsletter of Well Spouse, is published bimonthly.

Eldercare Locator
800-677-1116
www.eldercare.gov

Funded by the Administration on Aging, the Eldercare Locator offers seniors and their caregivers a national directory of local support services and resources.

The Simon Foundation for Continence
P.O. Box 815
Wilmette, IL 60091
800-237-4666
www.simonfoundation.org

The Simon Foundation for Continence offers information and support for individuals with incontinence, as well as their families and the health professionals who provide their care. The foundation provides books, pamphlets, tapes, self-help groups, and other resources. It does not provide incontinence supplies or funds to purchase them.

SUGGESTED READINGS AND PUBLICATIONS

Numerous publications are available that can be helpful in understanding more about memory disorders and caregiving and that offer additional activities and programs for memory-challenged individuals. This list is by no means exhaustive, and we suggest that you also look at the always-growing number of books on Alzheimer disease and related disorders to see what is available that will best address your concerns and needs. You can find most of the books listed below through your local library or bookstore or online bookstore.

At the Crossroads: A Guide to Alzheimer's Disease, Dementia and Driving
The Hartford, 2000
www.thehartford.com/alzheimers/brochure/html

This booklet can be downloaded from the above site for free. It is a guide to help the caregiver determine when it is no longer safe for a loved one to drive, and it offers support and advice for following through on that decision when it becomes necessary.

Bell, V., Troxel, D., Cox, T. M., et al.
The Best Friends Book of Alzheimer's Activities
Health Professions Press, 2004

This classic book provides a wide range of activities for memory-challenged individuals and their caregivers that can be adapted for home or community care settings.

Camp, C., ed.
Montessori-Based Activities for Persons with Dementia
Menorah Park Center for Senior Living, 1999

This manual, edited by a researcher in the behavioral treatments of Alzheimer disease, describes activities that can be done in a group setting or on an individualized basis, such as simple craft projects or reminiscence activities. The book is primarily aimed at staff working in dementia care facilities, but with some modifications it can be implemented by the caregiver at home.

Grollman, E. A., and Kosik, K. S.
When Someone You Love Has Alzheimer's Disease: The Caregiver's Journey
Boston: Beacon Press, 1996

Written by a caregiver, this book provides information on the emotional issues experienced while caring for someone with Alzheimer disease.

Gruetzner, H.
Alzheimer's: A Caregiver's Guide and Sourcebook
New York: Wiley, 2001

This guidebook gives the caregiver easy-to-understand information on the course of Alzheimer disease and ways to cope with the challenging demands of caring for someone who has the disease.

Mace, N. L., and Rabins, P. V.
The 36-Hour Day: A Family Guide to Caring for Persons with Alzheimer Disease, Other Dementias, and Memory Loss in Later Life, fourth edition
Baltimore: Johns Hopkins University Press, 2006

This book is a classic text that offers information on all aspects of caring for a loved one with dementia. It covers information on the disease process, living arrangements, financial and legal considerations, daily care, medications, research, mood changes, sexual behavior, etc.

Mittelman, M. S.
The Alzheimer's Health Care Handbook: How to Get the Best Medical Care for Your Relative with Alzheimer's Disease, In and Out of the Hospital
New York: Marlowe & Co., 2003

Knowing the steps to take to get good medical care for some who has Alzheimer disease is important. Written by an expert on care management for the people with memory disorders, this book takes you through the processes of securing routine care and preparing for hospitalization. It discusses the role of the caregiver and gives points to think about when making end of life decisions.

Robinson, A., Spencer, B., and White, L.
Understanding Difficult Behaviors: Some Practical Suggestions for Coping with Alzheimer's Disease and Related Illness
Ypsilanti, MI: Eastern Michigan University, Alzheimer's Education Program, 1999

This is a manual that provides information on the various behaviors and problems that occur throughout the Alzheimer disease process, such as wandering, incontinence, agitation, resistance to care and impediments to activities of daily living.

Zgola, J. M.
Care That Works: A Relationship Approach to Persons with Dementia
Baltimore: Johns Hopkins University Press, 1999

This book focuses on how the caregiver can strengthen relationships and provide good communication with a loved on both at home and in a long-term care setting.

CRAFT RESOURCES

Most of the craft and activity products recommended in this book can easily be found at your local craft store. Additional suppliers for these craft products are:

S and S Crafts
P.O. Box 513
Colchester, CT 06415

This craft retailer has a large selection of arts and crafts supplies. You can request their catalog and place orders either through their website (www.ssww.com) or by phone (800-243-9232).

Attainment Company
P.O. Box 930106
Verona, WI 53593

This company specializes in products for children and adults with special needs. You can request their catalog and place orders either through their website (www.attainmentcompany .com) or by phone (800-327-4269).

~ ABOUT THE AUTHORS ~

CYNTHIA R. GREEN, Ph.D., is a psychologist with nationally recognized expertise in memory and brain health. She is the author of *Total Memory Workout: Eight Easy Steps to Maximum Memory Fitness* (Bantam, 1999), a critically acclaimed guide to memory wellness. Dr. Green lectures extensively on memory and related topics. Since 1990 she has served on the faculty of the Mount Sinai School of Medicine and the Mount Sinai Health System, where she is an assistant clinical professor in the Department of Psychiatry. Dr. Green has held various positions within the Mount Sinai Alzheimer's Disease Research Center, including co-principal investigator on several Alzheimer disease clinical treatment trials, and has published several professional articles on the subject. She serves on the Scientific Review Board of the Institute for the Study of Aging, part of the Alzheimer's Drug Discovery Foundation. Dr. Green is the president of Memory Arts, LLC (www.memoryarts.com), a company that provides memory and brain health training to organizations, corporations, and individuals.

JOAN BELOFF is a specialist in the field of gerontology, with more than thirty years of experience. Ms. Beloff serves as both the New Vitality program and community outreach director for Chilton Memorial Hospital, in Pompton Plains, New Jersey. She served as nominations chairperson for the National Association of Activity Professionals, Eastern Region and is a past president of the Society on Aging of New Jersey. Ms. Beloff has been honored for her innovative educational programs by the Catalyst Institute for Innovation and Excellence and by the Wayne Alliance for the Prevention of Drug and Alcohol Abuse. Ms. Beloff has published articles in *Spectrum Nursing* magazine and serves as editorial advisor for the *Elderly Health Services Newsletter*.

Both Dr. Green and Ms. Beloff regularly present at national conferences on aging and senior health. They have collaborated for many years on programs addressing memory wellness and senior health issues. They recently received jointly the New Jersey Partners for Success award from the New Jersey Partners in Aging, Mental Health and Substance Abuse for their innovative program on memory and alcohol abuse, "Keep Your Memory Sharp! Tips for Success."